This book is dedicated to all my sponsors. A deep bow of gratitude to the following: Cal Clements, Jeremy Ayers, Noah Sanders, Sarah Wright, John Rogers, Tamar Smidt, Willow Tracy, Betsy and Blair Dorminey, Don Young, William Addison, Pongsakorn Suppakittpaisarn, Pindi Arora, and Neal Anderson. May that inner peace always be with us, everywhere we step foot on earth.

Om shanti shanti shanti

TABLE OF CONTENTS

48

FOREWORD
By Cal Clements

I can testify to the overall veracity of Jacob Ogletree's account. He is one of those exciting people, the ones who are not satisfied to take life on its own terms. Every time you bump into him he has a new plan. I like that spirit. It is aggravating to sustain while it is in you, but when it is gone you miss it. Jacob's flavor, through all the vagaries, maintained an "up" quality. If you told him, "You've done a terrible thing here," he'd say, "Hey, you're right. So true. But I'm a new man today." Mostly, he didn't do terrible things. He did fun things. Funny things. Really, in my view, he ought to be a clown.

You may be thinking to yourself, "Gosh, this is a horrible introduction. I'm being told the author is a clown. I hate clowns. Moreover, Donald Trump is a clown. I might as well put this book down now."

Immediately, I feel I need to explain things and rehabilitate the character of the good Jacob Ogletree. To do so, we must look at the notion of lineage, the Golden Chain, the flow of glowing energy that passes from person to person. In yoga, a big deal is made of lineage. There's a story of a fellow walking along a river. He meets another fellow who just came from a temple. He asks, "Who is your guru?" The first fellow thinks about it for a while and then replies, "I don't have one." The other fellow starts to run off. The first fellow says, "Hey, where are you going?" The second fellow says, "Back to the temple. I've got to bathe all over again." It is the idea that if you don't have a teacher you are unclean.

As for me, I run a yoga studio in Athens, Ga. I've taught thousands of hours of yoga classes and quite a few yoga teacher trainings. So you might say that I'm a teacher, a guru, or even (according to a detractor of mine) a cult leader. But really I'm a clown. Or, more precisely, I'm someone who dreams of being a clown. I love clowns. Even the ones with grease paint on their faces. What I hate is the horror clowns. That's such a sad inversion of the meaning--rather like baby dolls that have been animated by the devil. Clowns are the expression of mischievous innocence, childhood wonder, and the grand feeling of being forever free. So, if you put on a costume and perform a show with that kind of spirit, you're a clown. If you do it all the time, whether there's an audience or not, you're a happy eccentric. Then if you add stretching to it, you have yoga.

My own teacher, Jeremy Ayers (1948-2016), was an eccentric who loved clowns and yoga. But Jeremy hated the idea of being a mentor, having students, or anything that was hierarchical. In his mind, we were all friends and artists. The idea was to inspire each other (not just one person inspiring everyone else). Recently on the radio someone asked him what he thought of being a cultural icon of Athens. He said that Athens was filled with cultural icons. Then he shouted, "Viva La Revolution!" So part of the teaching that I got from Jeremy was to avoid the linear, the lineage, the straight lines. Instead, go round! Revolve! Revolt!

Nonetheless, when you step back from the quotidian part of living and look at the overall story from a perch high above, like an eagle (or a vulture), it becomes clear that we have certain highly influential teachers. Their ideas stick. They go inside. They become who you are. Jeremy was that person for me. But who was Jeremy's teacher? Now that is open to wild speculation because he would never tell you. He'd protest, "All of the world teaches me: The living, the dead, the writers, the singers, the drummers, the animals. Especially the animals. And the plants. The soil. The seasons." Then if you pushed him, which you really wouldn't do, he might admit to the influence of his mother and father. Both wonderful people. Really into health, ethics, and civic duty. If you suggested Andy Warhol or Dali and surrealism, he would have none of it. He'd say that the magic happens among the anonymous and it is happening right now. In fact, in his mind, the past had dissipated, like smoke. You can no longer see it. You can't touch it. Maybe you can get a whiff of it. But isn't clean air better?

So that was my teacher. And now off we go to Jacob's book. I hope that you've gotten a new sense of the idea of clown and how it is a good thing to suggest that Jacob ought to count himself among their ranks.

INTRODUCTION: WHAT IS A YOGI RESIDENCY?

yo·gi

'yōgē/

Noun

1. A person who is proficient in yoga.

There have always been renouncers: men and women who leave the household stage, abandon the conventional life and wander around the mountains and forests to live a life of ecstasy. These men and women are called yogis and yoginis and their whole lives are dedicated to seeking oneness with God. But what is the purpose of yoga? Why has it become so popular today? It is a sacred science of knowing the inner dimensions of the self, the "atman" or soul.

Three thousand years before Christ was born, the Rishis contemplated the nature of the breath, of life and death, and of man's purpose on earth. Living in the Himalayas, these mystics kept holy ash on their bodies, had unkempt hair and took vows of poverty. The origins of yoga are so ancient that the yogis were called "necked philosophers" by the Greeks. Alexander the Great met yogis when he invaded India in 326 BCE. He was so impressed upon meeting these yogis that he brought a yogi back to Persia to be an advisor. In India, Alexander the Great (or his representative Onesicritus) had an interview with the Brahman sages, who lived near Taxila. One of these people, a man named Calanus (Indian

Kalyana), followed the conqueror to the west, where he died. The story of the interview and the story of the death of Calanus are described in several sources, such as the Anabasis by the Greek author Arrian of Nicomedia.

Around this time there lived the great sage Sri Patañjali. During his life of prayer and practice, Patañjali compiled and outlined the science of yoga, giving it a body with eight limbs. Today we know these limbs as the eight limbs of "Ashtanga Yoga," which date back as far as 400 CE. It touches me to see that someone who never left India and lived a dedicated life to God is still remembered, studied, practiced and lived. To me, this is the teaching itself. Patañjali's Yoga Sutras have now been translated into multiple languages and have spread to reach every corner of the world, influencing millions—including myself thousands of years later in Athens, Georgia, of all places.

Some historians speculate on the exact dates of Patañjali's birth and death (Patañjali is also depicted in Hinduism as having a thousand radiant white heads). While we don't know the exact years Patañjali lived, we do know that he succeeded in organizing Yogic knowledge into the eightfold path of Ashtanga. *Ashtanga* simply means "eight limbs" (ashta=eight, anga=limb). Together they form the *Pātañjalayogaśāstra*, which is one of the foundations of classical yoga philosophy of Hinduism.

In Sanskrit, *sutra* means "thread." The Yoga Sutras are broken down into four parts. The first is the portion of contemplation (*Samadhi Pada*), then the portion of practice (*Sadhana Pada*), then the portion of accomplishment (*Vibhuti*

Pada), and finally the portion of liberation (*Kaivalya Pada*). The Yoga Sutras should be studied, but not with just the mind, where they are only intellectually understood. They should be studied and practiced with the heart, which can then transform the whole self and universe. The sutras are always there, with the practitioner. It is the yogi's bible, always with him until the day he becomes the living sutra.

There are millions of people all over the world who get up every morning and recite the Bible, Koran, or Bhagavad Gita. They have recited these holy verses hundreds if not thousands of times. Why? Is it just to do it? No, it is because the Word itself is living and breathing. The Word uplifts and the Word illuminates. That is why understanding the philosophy of the Yoga Sutras and its daily application is of the utmost importance for the practitioner. Remember, spiritual perfection should not just be intellectually understood in your head, but felt and experienced in your heart.

Yoga has changed the course of my life in ways I never could have imagined. My prayers were answered when I called out to God seeking the way out of the darkness and despair of my ignorance, out of the unnecessary pain and suffering I was causing myself, and ultimately, out of my Ego and selfishness and into my heart and peace. It was that day that I turned to the light of yoga. I pray that you can tame the mind and its thoughts through the withdrawing of the senses (*pratyahara*). Little by little, we can train the mind. Through concentration (*dhyana*) the mind gets strong. Even in mantra repetition, the mind becomes focused and calm.

Make your mind beautiful and you will not need cosmetic beauty, for you will have cosmic beauty.

res·i·den·cy

ˈrez(ə)dənsē/

Noun

1. The fact of living in a place.
2. A residential post held by a writer, musician, or artist, typically for teaching purposes.

A residency is most commonly associated to the medical field and follows graduation from a medical program or school. We've all heard the term "resident physician" before, so I thought, "If there can be a resident physician, there can also be a resident yogi." Surely the world could benefit from such a residency. My "Yogi Residency" was essentially a unique, creative, and unconventional way of maintaining yoga at the center of my life while continuing my studies of the breath and the science of yoga following my graduation from the Yoga Teacher Training certificate program "Adventure Club!" held by Cal Clements, the founder of Rubber Soul Yoga Revolution in Athens, Georgia.

Cal was without a doubt my first physical guru. You know the saying, "When the student is ready the teacher will appear." Well, I can definitely attest that Cal "appeared." He was also the catalyst for me going vegan. Cal showed up for me every day, patiently giving me gentle (and sometimes stern) encouragement. He taught me the ancient art of clowning and creating space for spontaneous jubilee, helping me become liberated from the bondages in my mind that stemmed from the darkness of ignorance. Cal provided a lot of shade when I was a young sapling and taught through example, exemplifying everything I aspired towards as a novice.

The Yogi Residency was a "harmonizing" of East and West. Later, after my residency was over, I would read a book titled *The Music of Life* by Hazrat Inayat Khan, founder of the Sufi Order in the West. This very idea of harmonizing East and West was the same request made to Hazrat by his guru. Hazrat was instructed to travel to the West, bringing with him Sufism so as to "harmonize" the two worlds. Hazrat was fond of saying that the scientist who climbs the mountain of knowledge finds the mystic already at the top, waiting for him. Other notable Western spiritual figureheads who have harmonized are Ram Dass, Pema Chödrön, Richard Freeman, Kofi Busia and Steve Ross. Some of the more current harmonizers are figures such as Kino, Rusty Wells, Sean Corn, David Life, Sharon Gannon and Rodney Yee. My responsibilities as a "Yogi in Resident" were to do away with the poisonous herb *samsara* (conditioned existence) and purify the mind to eliminate disease and illness. Imagine what that world might look like. It would certainly be a heavenly place.

Jacob Ogletree

CHAPTER 1: GETTING CANNED

"The fool who persists in his folly will become wise."
—William Blake

Once upon a time many moons ago I was unpoetically fired from my job as a research lab technician at the University of Georgia's botany greenhouses. Long story short, I thought I could get away with skipping out on some watering duties one Sunday. The four employees, including my boss Michael Boyd, would rotate who was to water the greenhouses over the weekend so we each only needed to do it once a month. It had been a long week, and a very hot and humid week, it being toward the end of summer in Georgia. My muscles were sore and I was tired. I just didn't want to cycle all the way out to the greenhouses that weekend. I managed to make it on Saturday, but not Sunday. The laziness had reached me. I made up an excuse for myself not to go by saying, "Well you know, I watered Friday and Saturday," and "Oh, look how cool and cloudy today is—the plants probably don't need much watering." Too bad my idea of a harmless skip day ended up not only costing me my job, but costing some research professors roughly 10,000 dollars' worth of research plants.

I did not react like a yogi. I was in shock, maybe even a little dumbfounded; definitely not at peace. I couldn't believe what had just happened. It was a real surprise for me. "Was I still fumbling in life?" I wondered to myself. "Wasn't I more mindful than that? Didn't I, Jacob Ogletree, practice *asteya*? Wasn't I a better yogi?" It stung. I didn't know how to process it all, so I just disappeared into the woods at the Georgia botanical gardens outside of town to be alone with myself and the trees in hopes of attaining some level of acceptance sitting by the river. I was confused and frustrated, sometimes crying, "How did you let one of the best jobs you've ever had slip through your fingers? What will become of you now?"

Looking back, I just laugh, because I can see with hindsight it was God helping me to turn within, towards Him. In fact, I was very fortunate in that respect. I was getting well roasted in the fires of *tapas*, becoming more refined. Nobody said getting refined was pleasant. We learn more from pain than we do from pleasure. I was afraid of what the future held for me because I didn't know what was next. I had no safety net: No family member was going to snap his or her fingers and bail me out or come to my rescue. I hadn't mastered the art of surrender, which is also known in yoga as *ishvara pranidhana*. I still thought that I was actually doing, instead of seeing God's invisible hand working through me, working through everything. I hadn't realized fully that God was already carrying me. In fact, He is already carrying the whole world. But at my novice stage, the money thing still affected me psychologically; I was afraid I would not be able to find the money I needed to survive. So really, we can trace the fear back to the fear of dying.

But it wasn't all doom and gloom on those long walks at the botanical garden. I also reminisced about the good times I had had working in the greenhouses. There were three greenhouses I was responsible for. The first of the three was the "primitive biome," full of cycads, which are one of the oldest families of plants. The cycads were once more abundant and diverse during the time before the dinosaurs roamed, but are still growing today, most commonly known as ferns and certain palm trees. I really liked the staghorn ferns that grew on the walls and the jade tree (crassula oveta). When you are in the cycad room, you get the impression you are in the land of the lost and you can almost imagine a pterodactyl flying over your head.

Next was the "desert biome," which was full of succulents and cactuses. Some cactuses touched the very roof of the greenhouse, which stood between twelve and fifteen feet tall. I've had a fondness for cacti my whole life. My earliest memory of a cactus was in the carport of my grandmother's house in Orlando, Florida. It should have been transplanted into a bigger pot years before. I would rub my palms up and down it and enjoy the prickly sensation. If one meditates on the cactus long enough, it will reveal to you all its secrets: the secret of retaining water and pulling water out of thin air just from breathing. Some cactuses are eaten in what is known as a peyote ceremony. Some bear edible fruits, "tuna" (as it's called in Mexico), a plump little fruit the size of a small peach with deep hues of purple and a mild fruity flavor full of edible seeds. Some cactuses are eaten in Latin American dishes known as "nopal." If you have just one cactus in your home, have the aloe vera cactus. The slimy flesh can be used to treat sunburns for the fair skinned and can also be used in smoothies to treat digestive issues.

The last of the greenhouses I was responsible for tending was the "tropical biome." Most of all, I remember the stillness in the mornings watering the orchids, birds of paradise, and begonias. The thick, heavy humid air was something familiar to my native Florida body and lungs. My first time eating passion fruit was in this greenhouse, when the ripened fruit would fall from the roof of the greenhouse. It tasted like a cross between a strawberry and a kiwi: very slimy and seedy, but oh so delicious. The rainforest greenhouse was where I would have my deepest and most profound moments and meditations listening to the soft rushing of the small waterfall, watching a frog leap off a lily pad and into the water. Plop…. There was no time, no rushing, no money, no taxes, no democracy, no politics, no religions and no judgments; just a quiet peacefulness that emerged from within and without.

It was a pleasant time for me. I was being uplifted by all the hues of green and the rich oxygenated environment of a glass house full of plants all exhaling oxygen. I was so inspired that I started taking cuttings of my favorite plants and working with rooting hormones. A lot of my cuttings took root and became their own trees. For those who don't know: Plants and trees are living fractals. To put it a little more simply, in every part of the tree there exists all the information needed to grow another tree without a seed. One's mind starts to drift into the beauty and symmetry of plants. I had my own little nursery going and seed bank. I started collecting a lot of seeds, mostly fruit seeds. I'd dry them out and save them from the farmer's markets, Whole

Foods or the Daily Co-Op. At one point I even planted a date palm in the desert biome, feeling more connected with arid climates.

During my time at the Georgia applied science greenhouses, I learned that no single seed is so weak that it needs to be planted in tilled soil. I learned about stratification. In horticulture, stratification is the process of treating stored or collected seed prior to sowing to simulate natural winter conditions that a seed must endure before germination (apple seeds are like this). Some seed species undergo an embryonic dormancy phase, and generally will not sprout until this dormancy is broken. When it was all said and done, I had grown to be more in touch with the plants while studying them. Put simply, they taught me how to grow.

After I was fired, I found a new job that was much less lucrative: stressing over what I was going to do next to earn a living. I was out walking one morning, not long after being fired, with my dear friend William Addison, getting things off my chest. I was a little emotionally unstable at times. This overwhelming sense of vulnerability loomed over me. I didn't know where to look or where to start. I was distraught at the thought of having to go back to working at a place like Buffalo Wild Wings, my first job in Athens. Thankfully, William was able to set my ass straight as we walked along the sidewalk. In his direct, yet sweet and nurturing tone, he said, "Jacob. The Sun, Moon, and Stars all have their best interests for you. You just can't see it yet. Accept that it will all manifest and be totally taken care of if you trust in your mantra. This is all for your benefit and for your education."

A few days after my walk with William, the Yogi Residency was born. I recall it today like it was just here and now. I was outside the Daily Co-Op, an organic food cooperative run by volunteers that supplies seasonal fruits and vegetables from local farmers. I was getting lunch with a longtime friend and artist, James Shepherd. Cal happened to be there (in a small college town you tend to run into each other often). It was warm and slightly muggy; sweat ran down my back and brow while outside enjoying a vegan bánh mi. I confessed or rather professed to the spondiferous Cal what had happened with me getting fired and that I might have to drop out of Adventure Club and live under a bridge. I rambled on about my fears and financial obligations. I was so concerned with things like rent, Yoga Teacher Training tuition, food and my phone bill.

I wonder how I must have looked and sounded to Cal. I am very fortunate to have had a loving, supportive guru like Cal. He was there for me in my lows and he was there especially in the highs. He just smiled and said, "Well Jacob, I've had the idea for some time now of having this kind of outlined program designed to separate oneself from capitalism 'temporarily' and to be fully immersed in an inquiry. There would be sponsors that supported you financially to help create a sort of bubble around you, shielding and protecting you from monetary distractions, creating space for magic to take place." Cal mentioned that he'd had the idea for a few years and at one point there was even a woman who was going to do the residency, but the opportunity didn't work out for all parties involved. I just knew right then and there that this was the idea I'd been waiting for. This was what I was going to do. My imagination was running wild.

I want to pause here and say that Cal was so good at dreaming, not just fanciful dreaming but artfully dreaming with articulation. One of the qualities I admired so much about Cal was that his level of play matched his self-mastery and discipline. After Cal finished, I told James I would meet back up with him later and ran home in excitement to break out my pen and paper and start rough drafting and laying out the foundation of the residency. After a few talks with Cal we settled on a good title, "The Yogi Residency." It had a nice ring to it. Something was definitely happening. I wasn't so afraid anymore, despite the obstacles still in front of me. Before the Yogi Residency could become a reality, I needed sponsors—ten to twelve to be exact. I didn't have any sponsors that day or the following week. I was living off food stamps and even sold my Adzuki road bike to pay rent for that month, but I had my imagination and my hopes and dreams to hold onto. I became excited and saw the future as less frightening and more ideal.

BREATHING EXERCISE #1: SURRENDER

- Inhale…and God approaches you.
- Hold the inhalation…and God remains with you.
- Exhale…and you approach God.
- Hold the exhalation. And surrender to God.

—Krishnamacharya

- Repeat this cycle with an inhale count of 5–10 seconds. Hold at the top of the inhalation and an exhale count twice as long as the inhale (10–20 seconds). Hold the exhale for 1–4 seconds. Repeat this cycle 10–15 times.

CHAPTER 2: LETTERS TO MY SPONSORS

"Your theory is crazy, but not crazy enough to be true."
—Niels Bohr

Around this time things get a little, how do I say, "phantasmagorical." Cal gave me the spiritual name "Felix." I began addressing myself to everyone as Felix for the next year. I'd say about a hundred or so people still address me and know me as Felix. My whole reality started bending and becoming distorted. New name, new personification: the Yogi Resident. As my surfer friends would say, "Far out man." Cal gave me the name probably because I was fond of wearing this black t-shirt with a white capital letter F on it, and one day at Rubber Soul after a yoga class, Cal just started introducing me to people as ffff-Felix. I laughed, Cal laughed, and we all laughed. I just started going along with it. I thought it was great, but after it stuck, I realized I didn't know the etymology of the word "Felix." I finally spoke up, "Hey Cal, you know I don't mind the new name. In fact, it's great and everything, but what does it mean?" He explained that the name Felix stems from the Roman cognomen meaning "lucky, successful" in Latin. The male version being Felix and the female version Felice. Both male and female names stem from the word "felicity," which is a noun for "intense happiness." There was something genuine in it. I was flattered and I did think of myself as rather a lucky fellow. It was an unforgettable time for me in the shaping of my character. Revisiting these pre-sponsorship letters are somewhat embarrassing, but in a good way. I was definitely all enthusiasm and spunk.

1ST LETTER: WRITTEN THE 15TH OF OCTOBER 2012

I Felix, otherwise known by my Christian born name "Jacob," would like to invite you to take part in an experimental residency program I have co-created with much help coming from professor Cal Clements. Residencies are an opportunity for an advanced training in a field of study, (mine pertaining to yoga and meditation). Often, you will see the word used in medical terminology, such as "resident physician." It is my sincere wish to renounce work for once and to observe a personal discipline of daily practices revolving around the betterment of planet earth and our species. My hope is that with enough sponsors I may sustain myself without the need for work and become more rooted in my Yogic Practices and dream. Here I've put together a list of my current expenses and cost of living:

RENT: $150
FOOD: $20
PHONE: $30

The total sum of my living expenses comes out evenly to two hundred dollars a month. This is the amount I need every month to 'get by.' As a sponsor your contribution is just $20 dollars a month. With just ten sponsors I can begin the residency. As a sponsor, you will also receive a weekly newsletter of how the residency is going. So, if you are indeed interested in participating in this experiment and are a supporter of Yoga and meditation and would like to contribute to the cause, then great! You will then have one of two payment options: 1.) Write a check for the whole six months $120 or 2.) Simply donate $20 every month to 670 West Broad St. Athens, GA 30601. For those who'd like to write a check, you may write it out to Jacob Ogletree. For those interested in contributing in other ways I accept all vegan food offerings. Again, it is my hope that with your support and sponsorship I may manifest the Yogi Residency program for the next six months and become solely immersed in this ancient art and science.

Warm hugs,
Felix

2ND LETTER: WRITTEN THE 21ST OF OCTOBER 2012

Greetings everyone!

Before we proceed I would like to give a standing applause to the following recipients for their contributions to the Yogi Residency Program thus far. John Rogers, please stand. Willow Meyers, please stand. Cal Clements, please stand. Sarah Wright, please stand (crowd applauding, and cheering). On behalf of every aspiring young yogi and yogini, I thank thee for making your contributions to this program! We are off to a great start; however, we are still seven sponsors away from the viability of the YRP. It is currently the 21st of October and the Yogi Residency will start on the 1st of November. I have meditated more on the outline of the residency and thought more on what kinds of daily activities are worth investigation for the betterment of humanity.

<u>STUDIES</u>

- Nutrition
- Food chemistry & biology
- Anatomy
- Conservation
- Sustainability
- Yoga
- Nature which includes earth, ecology, the four seasons, the solar system, the galaxy, and the universe alongside physics and astronomy
- Community building by being involved with the Athens farmers market, and S.O.S a UGA founded organization "speak out for species" and other activism.
- Adventure Club studies

<u>SADHANA</u>

- Meditation am/pm
- Cleanings (that consist of space and body)

- Prayer
- Gratitude notebook
- Breath work

SPIRITUAL ACTIVITIES

- Writing of poetry and prose
- Music playing (listening and practicing)
- Readings of spiritual scripture (that includes Hindu, Zen, Buddhism, etc.)

Sincerely,

Jacob Ogletree also known as Felix my feline incarnation!

I wrote everyone I knew who I thought would like to participate. I'm so glad I did. Granted, I remember thinking that 200 dollars a month was pretty cheap and could I really get by with that little? Then I reminded myself that yogis live on no money at all, with just a little more than what they had when they came into the world. By all the stars in heaven, I got all ten sponsors to sign up before November 1st. The entire three weeks leading up to the start of the Yogi Residency was a constant internal dialog: "Is this going to work? Am I really about to do this?"

My sponsors ranged in age, race, and careers. Cal helped out at Rubber Soul by pitching the idea to potential sponsors and served as a sponsor himself. Betsy and Blair

Dorminey were lawyers. Willow Tracy was also a lawyer. John Rogers was an electrician and landlord turned yogi. Noah Sanders, who I had a romantic love affair with, and the now late Jeremy Ayers were two of the most notable artists in Athens (ok, I can't leave out Terry Rowlett). Pongsakorn Suppakittpaisarn and Tamar Smidt were roommates at Ben's Bikes and students at UGA. Pindi Arora was a close friend and lover (I made a lot of love in Athens, what can I say?) who delivered handmade and blessed Indian dishes once a week, the recipes of which were taught to her by her grandmother in India. William Addison was a sponsor and on my support team cheering me on. Neil Anderson was a Rolf Zen master. Don Young was my landlord who probably pitied me. Sarah Wright was a professor at UGA and a close friend of Noah's, who thought that the Yogi Residency was something worthwhile and wanted to contribute. All in all, it came together. I still wonder how it happened. It was a pipedream. I should have gone back to washing dishes in a restaurant, but I didn't. I became the first sponsored Yogi in Resident.

Let this be a lesson to anyone out there looking for a way in. It came for me in the form of the Yogi Residency and it can come for you in the form of a Yogi Residency too! Nobody wrote the book on it until I did, and by this I mean that nobody has the right to say what can and cannot be done. Look around you, look at history, and look up at night. I think that everything in existence has been given approval and a big "yes" from God. So start saying yes to yourself, your big ideas, imagination and dreams. Have some fun!

BREATHING EXERCISE #2: LIGHT BODY

- Close your eyes. Focus your attention on your breathing. Focus on the air coming in through the nostrils, slowly and deeply, exhaling also through the nostrils. Let each breath come in a little deeper than the previous inhalation and each exhale go a little slower out of the body than the previous exhale and more completely. Repeat this ten times.

- You can also visualize breathing in a white light that fills your body and purifies. When exhaling, imagine breathing out a thick, black smoke. Repeat this inhale–exhale pattern until your whole body is filled with a divine white light. Then, you will no longer identify with your physical body. Not its shape, weight, or the color of your skin. You will just identify with the light.

Jacob Ogletree

CHAPTER 3: ADVENTURE CLUB

"Even the smallest person can change the course of the
world."
—Cal Clements

I first moved to Athens, Georgia with my good friend
James Shepherd in a 1994 Ford Thunderbird, our two guitars
and 400 dollars in cash along with a dream that we were
going to make it as musicians and become the next R.E.M.
When we first moved to Athens it was a rodeo. We had no
place to stay and we didn't know anyone—we were totally
throwing ourselves into it with no plan. I kid you not: our
first night in Athens I got drunk on a bottle of wine on the
UGA campus, rung the bell, ate a burrito and ended up
sleeping in the car behind the Crimson Cafe just outside of
Athens in Watkinsville, Georgia. For a few nights we camped
behind the women's soccer field, but the cops were always
around and we didn't think it was the right place. We finally
pitched our mobile sanctuary behind Athica, an old brick
industrial building turned art gallery. I remember this tree
growing inside this sort of courtyard of one of the buildings.
We slept in a two-person tent on a grassy slope leading down
to the train tracks.

Wandering sadhus, bum musicians, artists and spiritual
aspirants we were. Never have I been woken by a train's
horn so many times at night in my life. But that didn't faze
us. We were so alive and smiling, laughing hysterically at each
other and the wonderful adventurous life we were living.

There's a real difference between existing and living. Life was novel and happening for the first time for me in two years. It was so rich, so exciting. It wasn't really even stressful with the threat of running out of money (we couldn't even fill the tank with gas) or the threat of getting our camping gear stolen by train bandits. Not in the least. We were just always laughing! We bathed in the Ocoee River at the Georgia Botanical Gardens with a bar of soap. I didn't realize I was already the yogi I was aspiring to be.

Eventually we managed to move out of the tent. James found employment at a Jimmy John's and rented out a basement room in a big yellow house. As for me, I was living the musician's life, still on my girlfriend Katherine Klimt's couch. (Yes, related to the artist Gustav Klimt, coincidentally a painter I've always been very fond of.) We eventually separated, and I found myself walking down Millage Avenue: The boy wonder with a suitcase full of his clothes, an acoustic guitar, a book, and a toothbrush, walking to James who I knew would put me up a couple of nights.

On my way to James's place I passed an old antebellum house on a side street. A voice called out to me: "Jacob? Is that you?" It was my good friend Marty Cronk, a director of cinematography and artist.

"Oh hi Marty, yeah it's me alright."

"What are you doing walking with that briefcase in your hand?"

"I'm moving."

"Come on in man, my landlord's a cool dude, he will probably put you up for a couple a days."

So like a good guest who is being served tea, I took my warm cup and walked in. It was a dark, candle-lit house smelling of old books. Classical music was playing on an old record player. At the far end of a long, dark corridor, a large man sat smoking a long, fat cigar in the dining room. A light cloud of blue smoke filled the dimly lit room. I introduced myself as a friend of Marty's and he replied in a bellowing, Victorian voice.

"Hello my dear boy! So Marty tells me you got kicked out on your ass now did you? Well then come! Come, come my dear boy; you have the choice of *this guest room* or *this guest room*!"

I chose to sleep in a room that was in the shape of an octagon, the same room in which his parents were wed. The man's name was Jeffrey Tate, but he liked to be addressed as Jeff. His father was the dean of the University of Georgia back in the 60's and they named the Tate Center or "student learning center" after his father's contributions to the university during the Civil Rights Movement. Jeff lived alone in the family estate that stretched back seven generations and rented out the right wing of the house to Marty and his girlfriend. Though he had kids, they never came around. I think he must have run everyone off. Jeff was a first chair trombone player and an exceptionally skilled chess player. He'd even won some international chess matches in Atlanta in his day. We'd play chess long into the night with Jeff laughing, telling story after story, smoking cigars, drinking wine. He was also fond of reading Tennessee Williams poems, especially "Gold Tooth Blues." What a fine gentleman! I am endowed to him.

Around the same time I moved in at Jeff's, I befriended a woman by the name of Gretchen Elsner, who would unintentionally help me find my house in Athens for the remaining two years I lived there. We first met outside the Daily Co-Op one evening. I bought a pop-up book she had written and handmade for her son and offered her some chocolate I had just bought. She was on a different trip than most. Gretchen lived out of a trailer that she was building by hand from the ground up to be 100 percent solar powered and net zero. She was a protector and voice for Mother Earth, riding a bike everywhere and showing up to protests with giant puppets to assert our need to reduce our carbon footprint.

My two-week invitation at Jeff's place was up. I mentioned to Gretchen that it was growing too cold to live outside, and asked her to keep me in mind if she heard of any rooms to rent. I asked her about going in on a place and splitting the rent since I had very little money. For the better half of my adult life, I have relied on miracles and never on what my outer circumstances may have looked like and definitely not on the odds (I was always outnumbered), but my blind faith would miraculously carry me farther than I could carry myself. Gretchen never moved in, but it was thanks to her I met Don Young, my soon-to-be landlord. I sold my scooter and paid Don 250 dollars for a single bedroom with cement floors, one window, and a small closet. I spent my first night in the room cleaning the floors and walls and feeling so grateful for the empty room. I would live there for two years. It was a real series of trials and tribulations getting to Athens, but it actually happened, despite the adversities and odds. And it proved to be one of my greatest accomplishments.

At 27, having practiced yoga for five years, I feel as though I'm only just beginning to touch the surface of the more subtle, finer vibrations of sound and light (two aspects of movement united by harmony) and becoming firmly rooted and established in all eight limbs of Ashtanga and the inner life—100 percent inner life and 100 percent outer life. The inner life is what the soul delights in and is where you find fulfillment. The outer is also important and needs attention and tending. I didn't always have a lot of peace. I did have a mind, but not a peaceful, tranquil mind or heart, or an experience of the music of the spheres. I was once a very lost soul clubbing the darkness to beat it away when all I needed was to light a candle. Notice how the darkness leaves without a word or putting up a fight at all as soon as you light the candle.

Like many angst-ridden youth labeled ADHD, I was unwilling to compromise, or for that matter do anything my parents or adults told me to do. I just had to question, like Aristotle said. My sense of independence needed to be felt. I was a rebellious, anti-establishment, punk skateboarder who graffitied trains in the middle of the night, trying to step over crack pipes and homeless, refusing to conform. I flunked out of school and ran away from home. Wow. I'm so glad I found the light. I was really lost. I didn't have any direction. I was running here and there. A lot of my friends were taking painkillers. Even some of my most talented and gifted friends were ending up as electricians or in jail. I had hit the proverbial "rock bottom" with a few broken bones.

I moved back to my mother's house in the middle of nowhere on a mountain in Tennessee for nearly two years. One day I came across a YouTube video titled, "You are not stuck." I clicked on it because I was feeling very, well, "stuck." As I watched this slow-speaking, white-bearded sadhu speak to me, I began to feel very easeful and entered into a relaxed and wakeful, peaceful state—the meditative state—maybe for the first time. All from listening to the voice of this "YouTube Sadhu." His message was simple: "matter is vaporous." That there is no substance to matter at all and that everything must change hence — "matter is vaporous." The video totally blissed me out. I looked into more videos by him trying to get back to that wakeful, peaceful meditative state by listening to his voice. When his voice no longer blissed me out it was time to learn to listen to the inner Guru Ji speak. I decided to learn how to meditate for the first time in my life at 19. I'm so grateful to have retained a sense of awe and wonder, innocence, play, and good heartedness through all those dark days. I am grateful that my life did not take a darker path. These days I feel like sharing all my gifts. If I can help brighten someone's day, then that is enough for me.

The first time I met Cal, he was alone at Rubber Soul. He was standing on a ladder hanging beautiful dark purple drapes he had made. I walked in unannounced and introduced myself. I asked Cal if he had ever heard of the idea that if you put 10,000 hours into something, say your craft or art form, you'd become the master of it. He just said, "Ah, yes, 10,000 hours, very good. But what about 20,000 hours? What then?" We both laughed. I thanked him for taking time to talk to me and left thinking, "Wow, that Cal guy is so cool. I want to go back there and take a yoga class with him."

After that first meeting, I suppose I was officially indoctrinated into the temple of yoga. Life became phantasmagorical for me from there on out. I started going to Rubber Soul regularly and putting 5 dollars in the donation box. I think my very first Yoga class prior to Rubber Soul was a drop-in at a studio next to Earth Fare in Little Five Points, a power lunch hour of vinyasa. I was so clueless. I didn't know any of the poses the instructor was calling out. My only prior exposure to yoga had been three Rodney Yee DVDs that I practiced at home (and that one drop-in class, of course).

Nothing could have prepared me for the joys of Athens, Georgia, the joys of Rubber Soul, and especially the joys of Adventure Club apprenticing under Cal. I only attended Cal's classes. I tried other instructors and other studios in town, but none of them had the master's touch. I began making friends and meeting all kinds of local characters from town. Practicing back-to-back, mat-to-mat. I remember classes sometimes would be so packed that everyone was literally mat-to-mat from front to back. Someone's foot would touch your head or your leg would extend out onto their mat and everyone would laugh. I set my mat at the back of the studio in the beginning and eventually worked my way to front and center. Rubber Soul attracted a whole host of open-minded, eccentric-eclectic-peaceful-healthy, and happy people. The biggest message one receives going to Rubber Soul is that you belong, in all your weirdness and glory. After about a year of regular attendance, I found out that the next year's Yoga Teacher Training, "Adventure Club," was coming up. (The "Adventure Club" Yoga Teacher Training Program is still held at Rubber Soul in Athens and I highly recommend it— http://www.rubbersoulyoga.com)

When I found out that graduation from that year's Yoga Teacher Training would coincidentally land on my birthday, I saw it as a sure sign to go ahead and sign up to become a Certified Yoga Instructor. It just made sense. I wanted to continue to deepen my understanding, deepen my practice. I was being pushed and pulled deeper into yoga. Devote your life to selfless service and you are a Yogic master. No certification required. I don't even know where my certificate is—long gone by now, lost in all the moves. It must have walked out happy and liberated. But yes, it is very useful to have a guru in the beginning to show you the ropes.

I passed Adventure Club with a D+. In my defense, it was very tough final exam. Adventure Club was designed to cover yoga and its branching limbs: anatomy, physiology, the Yogic diet, what it means to be a vegan, nutrition, the eight limbs of Ashtanga Yoga, meditation, poetry, and some theater. There were quizzes and exams coupled with documentaries to watch and books to read and review. Our syllabus included the following: *Healthy at 100*, *Green for life*, the *Bhagavad Gita*, *Happy Yoga*, *Slaughter House* and *Eat to Live*. We met once a week for an entire day: 12 hours, 4 weeks a month, for 4 months. Those were marathons of days. Full of play, study, and yoga, yoga, yoga! It's where I started my journey in not just living but thriving off a plant-based diet and going vegan. We always prepared and ate meals together, walked together, played together, and studied together. I remember dancing with a towel in front of a mirror for nearly 45 minutes and then being blindfolded and lead around for another half an hour. Then being seated and having my feet dipped in a bowl of warm water while getting a foot massage. Long days working with the same pose over and over on alignment, posterior, anterior, extension, contraction. Adventure Club, what a fitting name! This all continued until the 8th of December, when we graduated from our 200-hour teacher training. It was a spectacular day. I turned 23 and life was wonderful. So take a vow then take a bow. Drop the curtains (your fear) and open your heart, into a field of infinite vibrational love.

Who is your guru? Who do you look to as your role model in your spiritual journey? Who embodies unconditional, universal love? Who radiates as vibrant as the sun and asks for nothing in return? Who is always peaceful and unaffected by external things? This is the person you should study and learn from as a spiritual seeker.

The guru's main purpose is to lead their student from the darkness of ignorance to the light of Truth. The guru can intoxicate you with their presence yet have an unexciting personality. They can put you in a blissful hypnotic trance state with their voice and words. Even then, only you and you alone are going to get up and practice every day on your mat and on your cushion or pillow without break, in all earnestness. That is the key to the transformative properties of yoga. It's also the part of the teaching that took me the longest to take to heart and understand. You will have days where you won't want to meditate or practice yoga and days where you have mediocre meditations and asanas. Do them anyway. I notice that in spirituality, people do not want discipline, yet there is discipline in schools and in work environments and institutions. So, why then is there not sacrifice and discipline in spirituality? There is great difficulty with a lot of seekers, for they come with preconceived ideas. They want to learn and are willing to learn but do not want discipline. Yet in the army there is discipline; in the factory there is a certain discipline; everywhere there is discipline. But in spiritual things, people don't want discipline; when it comes to spirituality they put up difficulties. They think so little of it and don't want to make any sacrifices because they don't know where it's leading to, they have no faith in God. There are false methods of spirituality taught here and people are commercializing that which is most sacred. The highest ideal is brought down to the lowest depth.

So and so may come and say, "Oh, I've been practicing yoga for years and I still haven't seen any changes." I then ask, "For how long? And has it been without break?" And they reply, "Well, off and on." See. That is why I say every day, without break. That is how you gain the supernatural powers (or *siddhis*) of the yogi. Look at Rusty Wells, Kino, Richard Freeman, Kofi Busia, Glenn Black, and Sean Corn. All of these teachers have something in common. They practice every day without break, in all earnestness. Patañjali mentions this in the second portion of Yoga Sutras (*Sadhana Pada*). Their transformations didn't happen overnight though. Everything in nature has its own time.

BREATHING EXERCISE #3: ALTERNATIVE NOSTRIL BREATHING (*NADI SHODHAN*)

Alternate nostril breathing is a wonderful breathing technique that keeps the mind calm, clean, balanced, happy and peaceful. It also helps release accumulated tension and fatigue. It only takes a few minutes. The breathing technique is named *Nadi Shodhan*, as it helps clear out blocked energy channels in the body, which in turn calms the mind.

- Sit comfortably upright with your spine erect, shoulders relaxed. A gentle smile on your face. Use your predominant hand and close the index finger and middle finger. You'll be using your thumb and ring finger and pinky.

- Close the left nostril and inhale through the right nostril. Close the right nostril and slowly exhale out your left nostril. Repeat this five times and then switch nostrils. After that cycle of alternate nostril breathing inhale through both nostrils and have a nice long exhale through the mouth with the tongue out; you can even make the exhale audible like fogging a mirror.

- After five repetitious rounds, you can just sit and breathe in and out through your nose regularly with eyes closed. Your meditation will be easier having balanced both hemispheres of the brain.

CHAPTER 4: THE YOGI RESIDENCY
NOV 1st, 2012 – APR 1st, 2013

"Know for sure that peace is worth more than anything else in this world."

—Sri Swami Satchidananda

I started the Yogi Residency program on November the 1st, 2012. I set my alarm clock for 5:00 am, and every morning before the sun, started with my pranayama and the opening invocation of Ashtanga:

OM

Vande Gurunam Caranaravinde

Sandarsita Svatma Sukhava Bodhe

Nih Sreyase Jangalikayamane

Samsara Halahala Mohasantyai

Abahu Purusakaram

Sankhacakrasi Dharinam

Sahasra Sirasam Svetam

Jacob Ogletree

Pranamami Patanjalim

OM

This translates as:

I worship

The supreme Guru

I bow to the lotus feet

At vision revealing true Self happiness

Knowledge

Beyond better (without comparison)

Jungle doctor conditioned existence

Poison

Peaceful resolution

All bodily limbs

Having the form of a man

Conch shell, wheel of light

Sword of discrimination 1,000

Headed

Brilliantly white I bow down

To Patañjali

After the opening invocation or prayer, I would begin saluting the sun—the sun salutations (*surya namaskara*) A and B. We salute the sun because the sun brings us life and we get the blessings of the sun God, that is why we salute the sun. Without the blessings of the sun we cannot be in full health. Then the six standing poses, all seated poses, all the vinyasas, and finally the finishing poses. It was very strenuous for me to not be panting and dripping sweat. It was difficult in the beginning; I would wake up so sore from the previous day's practice. I remember my hamstrings and hips were so stiff that dandasana was hard. I had to bend my knees so much to take the strain out of my lower back and touch my nose to my knees. But it got easier with time. I practiced on cold mornings on the cement floor in my basement room on my mat while frost blanketed the grass outside my window in the dim morning hours. Not even the space heater would warm the room some mornings. I'd have to crawl into an old military sleeping bag to keep warm. The cold air stung my throat and filled my lungs. Some parts of the Yogi Residency I absolutely don't miss. And some I do.

Once I finished my morning sadhana, I'd shower, brush my teeth, and walk to the Daily Co-Op for a cup of coffee and to write in my gratitude journal. I wrote all the things I was grateful for one by one for ten minutes to keep myself in the state of receiving and keeping the mind's attention on what I did have. In our Western society, we are conditioned to think we always need the newest thing, or simply the things we don't yet have. My gratitude journal was so effective I never ran out of things to be grateful for! I'm especially grateful if you're reading this line. In a way, I fantasized the Yogi Residency. Once I was in the full swing of Yogic practice, it was rather plain to the outside eye. Simple and repetitive with no variations. It became a meditation in and of itself—getting into the repetition of the same things every day in the same order. However, it wasn't boring.

After my hot cup of coffee and jazzed on caffeine, I was off to the main library on the UGA campus to study between three and four hours. It was very unconventional for me—hitting the books hard, spending an average of four hours a day for six months at the library, all while never officially enrolled as a student at UGA. I did sit in on a few physics lectures just for the pure enjoyment of it. I also sat in on Cal's comparative literature class one semester. Despite my unconventional methods, it worked. I already knew I was a bit eccentric and open-minded, and that traditional schooling and education wasn't for me. It didn't seem to make any real impression on me. I wanted to bypass the same old route I saw so many taking.

I had my passion for learning, growing and understanding and that's all I needed. I love to learn. The moment we stop learning we stop growing. I wanted to understand and master my breath, nature, my mind and my body. There should be more of these non-conventional schools in existence for the off-branch people like me that don't fit into the pretty little boxes and end up getting labeled as misfits. Even my attempts at college felt uncomfortable. Society tells everyone to go to college or they'll wind up working at a gas station. I knew I was going somewhere a little different on the path I was paving, though at times I was not exactly sure where. It was an intuition, a gut feeling.

After my four-hour sessions at the library, I'd make my way home merrily for a delicious smoothie made with the Vitamix (my favorite blender) that I had bought with some of my student loans. Usually something green and alkalizing! Victoria Boutenko's book *Green for Life* had a whole list of smoothie recipes in the glossary that I experimented with daily. I had ordered her book on a whim. What a whimsically good idea it turned out to be. The book offered a wealth of information and more importantly inspiration. One must empower the self with proper knowledge and wisdom of nutrition, food chemistry, human biology, anatomy, and diet if he/she is to reach optimal health and peak performance. We must also look at the subject from its multiple angles in the quest for health. I needed to educate myself about things like soluble and insoluble fiber, chlorophyll, alkalinity within the body, acidity, and how acidic environments are the breeding grounds for illness and disease. Victoria was an exceptional student of plants. She was the first person to get me really excited about edible weeds like dandelions, lamb's quarters and stinging nettle (a powerful liver and blood cleanser). A big tip for all you kale lovers out there that I picked up from Victoria's book: rotate your greens. There's a large variety of green leafy vegetables, and for every climate.

After my smoothie, I'd have an hour or two of leisure time where I'd take a catnap or meditate. At about 5:30 pm, I'd head over to Rubber Soul for another yoga class, which could spiral into clowning or band rehearsal or tea and stories or dinner. I've got to say, being a Yogi in Resident is pretty awesome. If you're reading this and wondering if you could do the same, let me just tell you, you can! If you're at a turning point in your life and ready for transformation, you can use the Yogi Residency as a template and platform for your own beautifully sculpted dreams. Take as little or as much from my story and strategy as you wish. If you think you'd like to start your own Yogi Residency, simply tailor it to your passions. You have more to gain than to lose by becoming not only a yogi or yogini in residence, but an example for what is possible to the world. There's so many ways to structure it and find benefactors or sponsors. Now there's crowdsourcing websites. A Yogi Residency's focus is always on union. Not on selfish gains.

I spent a lot of time in, out, and around Rubber Soul, as expected, those six months practicing asana with my guru—a lot of clowning too, mostly clowning actually. The boss clown Cal would pick me up, pick out a costume and an idea for a street performance and drop me off downtown in a pink leotard with juggling balls, or in a skunk outfit with a basket of wild flowers we'd picked in Jeremy Ayers garden. I was to participate in all rehearsals in our little clown troupe, The Hobohemians. We were a tramp clown troupe (say that five times fast!) in a band together called the Terrible Tuba Band. We were so terrible! We would all get into our stitches, put our makeup on, and load up into the back of an old Model T Ford Cal owned and ride up to a busy street corner on a weekend night. Simultaneously jumping out of the clown mobile, there'd be a little introduction and scripted words for our opening, followed by fantastic, spontaneous improvisation.

We'd address the audience and introduce our troupe, talk a little and then go into a number, "Somewhere Over the Rainbow," all on tubas. I loved to dress up as the British police officer and ride around on a tiny bicycle playing the constable character who was trying to stop the tramp clowns from entertaining the audience and prevent them from having fun. I loved it if the audience got so into it that they'd throw fruit or vegetables at me (luckily no beer bottles were thrown). I also marched in a marching band formed by Cal, playing the saxophone that was on loan to me from Cal. The marching band was called 350 Parts Per Million. We marched and played tunes like "When the Saints Go Marching In" all to raise awareness about global warming and what everyone can do to reduce their carbon footprint on the individual scale. Which is, as it turns out, to go vegan! It's the single greatest thing one can do to reduce their carbon footprint. "Fight global warming with your fork!" was our tagline. Good grief I loved that time with all my heart. I'd like to work my way back into that lifestyle and service to humanity in good time. It makes me very happy to reflect back on how wonderfully wild I was and see how much crusading and clowning I was doing at that time in my life for world peace.

I thought there might be more to say about the six months of the Yogi Residency. It was pretty consistent with all its daily activities, routines, and with all the clowning and such. I'd like to just say that creating all that time for me was one of the best things I've ever done for myself. Thanks to the seed thought from Cal and my craziness in believing enough to plant the seed and water it, I was spared from the jaws of mediocrity. I was protected in my bubble that my sponsors helped form. My miracle came in the form of the Yogi Residency, and anyone can do this. If you're holding this book or reading the eBook, it's because someone believed in a dream. You may be reading this for a reason, not just the mere entertainment of it. I believe you're about to do something pretty awesome. There are no coincidences. But it doesn't end there. At the end of the day, a residency is just an advanced study in a field. We are looking for something much higher. We are looking for the highest ideal. It's nice to study and practice, but we need to become masters. There is a certain level of sacrifice to be the master, but the process is very much worth the reward. The tallest mountain in the world is Mt. Everest, but as a spiritual seeker on the endless road to Spiritville, we are climbing an even greater mountain…Mt. Ever-Rest. May you find it within and find it here, right now.

Om shanti shanti shanti

BREATHING EXERCISE #4: BREATH MUTHAFUCKA!

This breathing exercise was first introduced to me as "birthing" and for good reason. I've seen it given a few other names but I like "birthing" because it's fitting and you'll know why soon enough. This breathing technique was taught to me by Cal during my Yoga Teacher Training, and was passed down to him by Steve Ross. Years later, I remember listening to a podcast with Wim Hof, the "ice man," who also practices this breathing technique and teaches his students, but using a different name for it.

- If you can manage to push through the barriers of fear and really not hold back and completely super oxygenate the bloodstream, it's a very alkalizing and powerful experience. I full on burst into tears my first time doing it, followed by hysterical laughing. Here we go, let's do it!
- Lie on your back, close your eyes, stick your tongue out and begin breathing deeply into the mouth and out of the mouth. Deep quick inhales and exhales. It

helps to have an upbeat motivational song to play. It'll help you keep your tempo of breathing. "Purple Haze" by Jimi Hendrix is a personal favorite. Keep this breathing up for 5–10 minutes, during which time you will start to feel a sensation come over you. Your whole body will start to tingle and your hands will start to close up. Your tongue will get dry like a lizard. When you finally stop your deep breathing, your whole body will be pulsating and vibrating. You won't even need to breath. Just feel. It's a remarkable experience. I still do it every month to reset. Don't be afraid—you won't die. It might feel like something crazy is happening, but surrender to that experience and enjoy it.

CHAPTER 5: WRAPPING IT UP— PRESENTATION TO MY SPONSORS

"I like nonsense; it wakes up the brain cells."

—Dr. Seuss

During the six months of the Yogi Residency, if you recall from the previous chapter, I went to the library every day to study my very own body of work. So what exactly was I was researching? Economics, sales, accounting? No. It was my thought that the best way to use the time I had been given was to create a clear understanding of the brain and meditation. It felt very important to me to see how health starts, in my opinion, with mental health.

I buried myself in books like some sort of postgrad student, compiling a hefty stack of research papers pertaining to meditation, the brain, neurology, neural oscillation, consciousness, matter and its application towards enlightenment from both Eastern and Western perspectives: from ancient wisdom to modern empirical science. With a little less than a month left in the Yogi Residency, I decided it was time to invite all my sponsors and friends over for a vegan potluck and presentation to reveal what I had learned. My gift was to present to my sponsors all I had learned during the last five months of investigation into the mind.

The bulk of my research for those five months pertained to the discovery of multiple underlying connections: the marriage of ancient wisdom on meditation to what modern science has to say about the study of the brain, how it works, and what happens to the brain during meditation. I wanted to flesh out what exactly was going on at different states of consciousness, from waking to sleeping to dreaming, and most importantly, during the meditative state. These were important questions to me and I was putting the puzzle pieces together. I wanted to use the knowledge I'd gained as a tool for expanding my horizons, educating not only myself but a greater audience on how freaking amazing our brains are and why we should meditate. If one only knew the power of meditation, one would not miss a single day or opportunity to sit.

My research dealt with higher states of consciousness ranging from beta to gamma to alpha waves, neurology and the study of how neurons wire and fire, neural oscillation, the single firing of a neuron and the firing of groups of neurons, the anatomy of the brain from the glands to the evolution of the human brain from the brainstem and cerebellum all the way to the seat of consciousness in the neocortex and prefrontal lobe. It's really too much to try and cram it all into this book, but it will all go into my next book on meditation.

I invited all my sponsors over for an evening of vegan cooking followed by an hour presentation on meditation and the brain. I borrowed a projector, a screen, and a friend's laptop. I looked for a VGA cable and put together the whole PowerPoint the day prior to the presentation. Don't worry, I won't leave you completely empty handed without a morsel. I'll give you a sneak peek into the outer mind's inner marvels.

For those seeking to dive deeper into meditation, its ability to change every aspect of your life for the absolute best, and the amazing capacity of your own brain, you will be able to get it all in my next book.

You do yourself no favors by not taking the time to understand the brain and how it works. The most common mistake made by people is putting self-limitations on one's capabilities and underestimating the true power of the human brain. If one could only understand a fraction of the capacity and creativity of the human brain that lies mostly untapped between your ears, you would not think anything is really impossible or out of reach. The mind is your best friend or your worst enemy. The mind also has a body and breaths of its own. We're so accustomed to identifying with our thoughts and brain, but after reading more on the brain you will begin to make the distinction and separation between the knowing of you and the thinking of you. You'll be more aware of yourself and your thoughts as a separate entity and know it's just the mind and not the actual you.

The brain is a dancing electric wave of patterns in three-dimensional space. Connected like a supercomputer and super sophisticated with close to 100 billion neurons, nearly equal to as many stars as there are in the Milky Way Galaxy, yet packed into a space infinitely smaller. But you don't have to think too hard: The simple Yogic answer is to just let thought become your beautiful lover by the depth and width of your breath. Our mind is deeply and directly connected to our breath. So much so, that if your breathing is shallow, so is the mind. If your breath is deep, so is the mind: calm and serene. How deep are you breathing right now? One must rise above the primitive mind of the limbic system and transcend even the prefrontal cortex to rise higher still through the breath out of the body, out of the mind, and into the highest gate of heaven.

I closed the presentation with a quote by a favorite mediator of mine, Thích Nhát Hanh: "As human beings, our deepest desire is to find an environment which is secure and where there is love and understanding. All of us want to live in such an environment. If you live in surroundings where you feel there is security, understanding, and love and where people have the capacity to transform their suffering, fear, and attachment, then you live in the Pure Land."

The pure land I interpret as the mastery of the mind. Once the mind is tamed, purified and the heart can be cultivated, then you are expressing the fullness of your highest self. You must first study and learn everything about the brain and mind to tame it, master it, and then simply to get out of it and into the heart. There are a billion rooms to live in in your mind: beautiful palaces in the sky and dark dungeon's underground. But the temple of love is seated in your heart. Live there.

My sponsors probably left with a feeling of expansiveness. I wanted to expand while also making the information accessible to a larger audience. I have to admit it was a beta testing presentation. Looking back and reflecting on my presentation, it may have sounded too academic because all the information hadn't settled. It was still so new to me that I hadn't had time to properly digest it and exude wisdom on the mind rather than regurgitating neurological jargon. Over the last six years, I've had plenty of time to log meditation hours and revisit my research papers. Mulling, musing and contemplating on the brain, allowing all the knowledge and wisdom to settle in. I am beginning to get the faintest notion that the Yogi Residency is going to be more valuable to the world than I ever realized. Hari Om!

BREATHING EXERCISE #5: MIND>MATTER

This exercise is just as much an exercise for manifestation as it is for breathing and mindfulness. The mind shapes matter. It's as simple as that. Thoughts become things. So with this breathing exercise, we're going to take a look at some sound vibrations and we're going to focus on what it is we want to bring about for us that are going to serve humanity and benefit the world. We need a clear precise vision of what it is we've always wanted. Not something small like a boat or a car or a house, though this exercise can work for manifesting those things to.

- Sit in an upright position. Close your eyes. Begin by focusing on your breath and bringing *prana* into your body. The two most creative centers in your body sit in the reproductive organs and at the seat of your third eye. Because the universe is polarized, we have opposites. Left arm, right arm. If you have hot water, you have cold water; if you have north, you have a south; if you have a head, you also have a tail, etc. This is the same with our creative centers. Within the sex organs, you have the semen or sacral fluids. Within them is stored all the creative energy to create life. A highly creative center given to us by the Lord that we mostly spill and waste. Most Westerners don't properly understand the potency of their seed. As you breathe in, you are going to focus on the base of the spine and send the sound "ahhh" into the base of the spine. This is the sound of creation. When a man and a woman come together to create new life the word "ahhh" is inevitably used during sex. So using this creative sound vibration we send it into the base of the spine. And moving the energy from there to the sex chakra, breathing in and exhaling the ahhh into it, then moving to the navel, ahhh, then to the heart chakra, breathing in and exhaling, ahhh. Moving the energy to the throat chakra, ahhh, then to the eyes, ahhh, then to the third eye, breathing in and again exhaling, ahhh, into the third eye, visualizing what it is you want to manifest and seeing it very clearly, and send the ahhh vibration into the vision and it cooks the thought like popcorn and aids in that vision manifesting into your experience. Then let it go. Ahhhh.

CHAPTER 6: FLYING TO OMEGA

In this dream world
We doze
And talk of dreams—
Dream, dream on,
As much as you wish
—Ryokan

As the Yogi Residency was drawing to a close, so too was my time in Athens, Georgia. I knew that it was time for me to take flight, spread my wings and fly. My two years in Athens was like one big, warm incubation. I knew that by the end of the Yogi Residency and with the coming of spring I would be ready to hatch and fly away.

I applied to live and work at two retreat centers for meditation and yoga. I wanted to continue my studies in the ways of the mystic and Yogic traditions. Six months of a Yogi Residency is good, but a lifetime of yoga is better. I applied for a seasonal position as an organic farm intern at Yogaville in Virginia, which was founded by Sri Swami Satchidananda and the Omega Institute for Holistic Studies in Rhinebeck, New York. These were the two ashrams (retreat centers) I settled on. I recommend any yogi or yogini seek out others on a similar path for support and accelerated growth.

William was the first person to ever tell me about the magical place called the Omega Institute. I could hear in William's voice that this was a special place that had left a beautiful watermark on his soul. William had been shown the Omega Institute through Anthony Flowers, who had done flower arrangements for the 14th Dalai Lama and Thích Nhất Hanh and Ram Dass. I feel like Anthony and the flowers were behind the scenes of my transformation. Anthony is also the author of *Being with Flowers*, a beautiful book on floral art as a spiritual practice. I have a lot to thank Anthony for—for opening the doorway for William, who in turn opened the door for me. And hopefully, I have now opened the door for you.

I remember William telling me a story one night about the time he had a glass of wine with Julia Butterfly Hill at Omega. He told me that after she left the room, he started crying. I was totally moved, since I had just finished reading Hill's book *The Legacy of Luna* in Cal's class. The book tells the story of her two-year journey living in a giant redwood tree to protect the redwoods from deforestation, a remarkably kind act that inspires me to this day to take a stronger stance on protecting the environment.

Later, I learned that Cal had also been to the Omega Institute and had taken a workshop with either Richard Freeman or Steve Ross. I was split between the two retreat centers—Swami Satchidananda was calling and so was Omega. So I decided that I would apply to both and accept whichever offered me a position first. I did just that. I applied to both Yogaville in Virginia and the Omega Institute in upstate New York and waited. About a week or two later, I heard back from Omega and arranged a Skype interview with Amina Eagle, who passed away shortly before publishing this book and whom I'd like to acknowledge as being one of the pillars of the Omega Institute since day one. I borrowed my good friend Elizabeth's laptop and set it up in the living room. During our conversation, Amina asked me questions that no one had ever asked me in an interview up to that point: "What do you love to do, Jacob? What makes your heart dance?" I was accustomed to, "What can you do for our company?" I told her that besides yoga, I loved to play music and that my father and my grandfather were musicians. She decided to put me in contact with Ken Kuter, director of the audiovisual department for Omega.

When I first spoke with Ken, he asked me what I played and how knowledgeable I was with mixing audio. I told him that I played the saxophone, guitar, and a little xylophone. I mentioned that I had run an XLR cable once in my life, and I was okay with operating the most basic four channel mixing board, but that I also was a (cough) quick learner by failing often and failing fast and that if there were any technical troubleshooting issues with the signal flow, I was positive I could figure it out. I swore I didn't need much training. I could hear in Ken's voice that he was a bit skeptical, wondering whether I was legit or completely full of it. He reminded me of all the responsibilities as an audiovisual technician: managing the audio decibel levels for PA for live kirtan, recording audio of workshops for archival purposes, all black dress code for large events, cables coiling and the rigging for lights, not to mention the annex. Ken probably only hired me because William was my reference.

I kissed Athens goodbye and stayed one night in

Atlanta at William's mother's house in Buckhead. The following morning William drove me to the airport. Whether or not I was ready, I was getting on the plane and heading for the mystery and adventure that would unfold. It really can be difficult, even scary to leave everything behind at the beginning of a pilgrimage to God. I even had a breakdown and a small anxiety attack in Atlanta the day before my flight. William, the angel he is, coached me through it. I was leaving behind the community I had been a part of for two years, the friends I had made, the familiarity of Athens (my security blanket and comfort zone). I didn't know when I'd return and if this all was even a good idea. But hindsight is 20/20 and I am very glad I went. When I got off the train in Rhinebeck from New York City, I had a huge traveler backpack and a guitar, but not enough money for the taxi to Omega. Luckily, two other girls (Ali Schmidt and Chelsea Mac, now my Omega sisters) were on the train heading to Omega and offered to split a taxi. I handed them my last 20 dollar bill and off we were to the enchanting and enlightening land of Omega.

I remember checking in with people and culture. They gave me all this paperwork to fill out and sign, took my picture, and said, "Okay, Felix" (I went that whole year as Felix), "now you get to pick one workshop for free, any workshop throughout the whole season. Some workshops are not allowed due to the length and some fill up fast, but go ahead and pick one." Flipping through the year's catalog, I remember thinking that I had hit the jackpot for all things spirituality (yoga, shamanism, dance, music, circus, and zen.)

I circled like twenty workshops including Alex Grey's visionary art workshop. I eventually narrowed it down to a Yin Yoga retreat: five days of Yin with Biff Mithoefer and his assistant Prema Mayi, whose devotional music and chants might be the best I've ever heard live.

I mean sure, I've had it rough, but damn, I've had it pretty good, too. Being backstage with Krishna Das, Skyping Ram Das live from Hawaii, listening to Pema Chödrön, singing along with Bobby McFerrin. Omega was like living in a karmic accelerator. I tear up just reminiscing sometimes. My love, Guru Rishi. Falling in Love with Meghan Meyer, who at the time was in the middle of her Jivamukti teacher training. My first time flying into New York City was so incredibly surreal. My biggest goal in life was to just make it to Athens, Georgia. Simple. I thought that when I finally got to Athens, I'd be there for at least ten years, but after two, I had become a clown's apprentice, Certified Yoga Instructor and was touching down in LaGuardia on my way to the Omega Institute.

My travels and the places I have gone were all just dreams dancing in my heart. Before I made it to Athens, I wanted to live in Colorado, California, New Orleans, and New York City once in my life. Seven years later, coming out of a meditation in Tulum, Mexico, it dawned on me that I had lived in all those places without realizing it. I had dream danced without fear seven years ago from my bedroom in Dunlap, Tennessee. If you asked me how I did it, I couldn't tell you. Only that deep down somewhere I believed. I didn't know how I would do it; I just dreamed it. I thought it could be done regardless of money or connections or resources or the notorious how-to instructional. That's something that makes me smile to reflect on. You have to believe in your dream, no matter how many times you fail—trust me. You're looking at an expert failure. No matter how impossible they say it is. No matter how much the odds are against you. You're going to do it. Dream on when others have stopped dreaming, even if you get shot down in mid-flight and have to start over from scratch. You might have to start over from scratch multiple times, but don't stop believing in your dream.

A good friend and teacher of a course in miracles, Erica Lee, once told me, "You know what I love about you Jacob? You're an authentic dreamer." Cal also pointed out something similar. He saw potential in me when I only vaguely displayed the desire to become a mystic, and he said that I had a natural gift at making people laugh and feel good and that I would make a decent clown. Maybe he was right.

BREATHING EXERCISE #6: OM SHANTI

- Sit in a comfortable cross-legged position. Sit tall, with an erect spine. Close your eyes. On your inhale silently draw in breath through the nose and visualize the sound vibration "om" traveling down your spine to the base of the spine, reaching the base of the spine at the top of the inhale. On the exhale, mentally exhale the vibration "shanti" as it travels up your spine to the crown of your head, entering the crown chakra. Repeat this visualization of the aaaauuuummmmm going in through the nostrils and down the spine and then the shhhaaannntttiiiii traveling up the spine on the exhale out the crown of the head until total well-being is felt throughout your whole body and mind.

The whole of creation is vibration. Scientists all tell us this. And so have the mystics. So your mantra generates a vibration, a frequency within you. A beautiful atmosphere will surround you and everything will totally be taken care of with your mantra alone. Know that spirituality is not what you are doing, but what you are thinking. Thoughts are the most powerful. Think of your mantra often. It is the simplest and most direct Yogic practice. Let your mantra become a part and parcel of your whole life, constantly coming back to it is watering. After a while, your mantra will always be repeating in you even when you are not thinking of it or saying it. It will be in your subconscious repeating itself. It will be in your heart and on your lips. All mantras are equally good. There is no better mantra than the other. They are all God's name. You don't even need to understand the meaning of the mantra, just repeat it, with feeling and without feeling. It is the simplest and easiest way to spiritual perfection. Many saints have attained enlightenment through their mantras alone. If you only have time for one practice let it be your Japa Yoga or mantra repetition. I was given the mantra by my guru "Hari Om." And "Om shanti shanti

shanti."

CONCLUSION: WHERE I AM

Listen: this world is the lunatic's sphere,
Don't always agree it's real,
Even with my feet upon it
And the postman knowing my door
My address is somewhere else.
—Hafiz

As the physicist reaches to grasp reality, reality slips through his fingers like sand. A beautiful analogy for this is in the study and observation of the electron. The electron sits in what is called a superposition orbiting the nucleus of the atom. At the quantum scale, particles can also be thought of as waves. Particles can exist in different states. For example, they can be in different positions, have different energies, or be moving at different speeds. But because quantum mechanics is weird, instead of thinking about a particle being in one state or changing between various states, particles are thought of as existing across all the possible states at the same time. It's a bit like lots of waves overlapping each other. This situation is known as a superposition of states. If you're thinking in terms of particles, it means a particle can be in two places at once. This doesn't make intuitive sense, but it's one of several strange realities of quantum physics. When the observer goes to look at the electron and shines light on the matter (pun intended), the electron assumes one of the many possible possibilities. Your whole life is the same. You are not meant to get it or to grasp it. You are meant to loosen the grip and to let *it* go and become one with all possible states. Become omnipresent.

The father of calculus, Sir Isaac Newton, said on his deathbed, "I don't know what I may seem to the world, but as to myself I seem to have been only like a boy playing on the seashore and diverting myself now and then in finding a smoother pebble or a prettier shell than the ordinary, whilst the great ocean of truth lay all undiscovered before me." What was Isaac Newton trying say with his last words? Despite his groundbreaking work and great achievements in his life, Newton was humbling himself before departure. To have discovered so much, yet still to know that an ocean of truth lay undiscovered. We all want to know the Truth. We all wish to touch the depths of our being.

As I sit and meditate on the Yogi Residency in all its glory and beauty, all of these things become just that: things. A greater sense of lightness is felt in my body. As my breath rises and falls, I release the bondages of attachment in my mind. Freeing myself from the bondages/attachments to people, places, things and outcomes so that I might rise more freely. Freeing myself of the attachment of how I wish it would be, how it could be, how it ought to be, and finally, allowing it to just *be* the way it simply *is*. Let your life just be the perfection that it already *is*, without judging it, for all the false notions of myself have burnt to ash as I near God.

In my meditations, I like to visualize my body as a living, breathing, and pulsating organism, imagining the stomach secreting its acids for digestion, or the billions of red blood cells carrying rich, fresh oxygen to the tissues, organs, glands and cells, focusing on the rhythm of the heart beat and the rising and falling of my breath. Imaging the heart with its intricate valves pumping this fresh, rich oxygen all over my body through the miles of veins and exhaling carbon dioxide gas. Seeing myself more as an electrical, pulsating, dynamic fluid body and gas than as a solid, static object. Still using my mind's eye, I go back in time to retrace the steps of my origins and evolution. I see myself wandering over the open plains of Africa, under the rain forest canopy swinging from branch to branch and swimming in the oceans. I let my thought become my beautiful lover as I rise towards God, and I feel infinite in expression without the need of a body or weight. I feel my DNA interconnected with all living beings.

I imagine the DNA in the nucleus of my cells and I feel its infinitely small, yet highly sophisticated and intelligent design. I travel past the mystery of the origins of life on earth, all the way back to when the iron in my blood was being forged in the heart of a dying star. We are, in the words of Carl Sagan, "star dust." I imagine myself at even more fundamental scales than the chemical or molecular scale, all the way to the atomic scale, 99.99999 percent of which is empty space and the remaining 0.0000001 percent pure energy. At this transcendental meditative state, one might even feel consciousness's effervescence. One might discover the mystery of life.

My investigations into physics, nature, and yoga have all shown me that things like particles, atoms, strings, black holes, stars, space, planets, dark matter, dark energy, plasma, plants, rivers, mountains, animals, yogis, and humans are all a part of a cosmic symphony and dance that's so amazing it can bring one to their knees weeping at its marvelousness. Even the particles spin in joy, all silently chanting His name.

If there is anything I've learned from yoga, it is what the scriptures have said from the beginning: "the kingdom of heaven is within." What that means is that everlasting happiness and peace is within. Once experienced, it does not change. Once we find happiness inside our hearts, there will be no more running. Then we are peaceful and joyful and we become better instruments of the divine. "First seek the kingdom of heaven and all shall be added unto you" (Luke 12:31). I've come to know this as the Truth.

There have been times in my life, including moving to Athens and just before the Yogi Residency, where I was at my breaking point, at the point of giving up, laying down and quitting. Even before these difficulties, I had mountains to climb. At that point, I raised my hands up towards the sky and called out to God, crying "I surrender Lord. It is out of my hands now. I give it all to you. I've done all I can do now. I can do no more. Do as you wish to me. I am in your hands now."

It was surrender—otherwise known in yoga as *isvara pranidhana* (pronounced "Ish-va-ra-pra-nid-hah-na"), the very last of the *niyamas* of Patañjali's Yoga Sutras. It was surrender that was my saving grace and which lies behind the Yogi Residency. It can be terribly frightening to let go and to surrender your pride, but you never lose what you give.

Suppose you give 100 percent to God. You get 100 percent *of* God. As Krishnamacharya once said, "Where is delusion when you know Truth? Where is disease when the mind is clear? Where is death when the breath is controlled? Therefore, surrender to Yoga."

However, if you wish to obtain success in yoga overnight, don't expect very much. If you are after someone or something on the material plane, you are after it day and night. You don't eat, you don't sleep; you are obsessed with it and always after it. If it takes that much focus and discipline to obtain little things on the surface like name or fame, what then does it take for success in spirituality and yoga? It takes a truly dedicated heart.

It also will take time. We Westerners don't want to hear this. We want it now. There's a joke about a man praying for patience and wanting it now. He wanted something small and a fast plan, so he planted a spinach seed and harvested it in thirty days. If you want something bigger and longer lasting, plant a fruit tree. It will take several years for the tree to even bear fruit. It will take time for the fruit to ripen and fall, and it will take time for the flower to bloom and produce fragrance. Everything has its own time, and we should not rush God's work and disturb our mind of its peace. Just let it come in God's time. Your body will continue to open and change through your daily asana practice.

We should not expect a smooth, problem-free ride either, as you can see from my own experience: the fiasco of getting into Athens, the fiasco of getting fired, and before those fiascos, I was a lost teenager with no guidance or direction. In a smooth, problem-free world, there would be no learning and no growing.

Now is the time to commit to yoga. Let our whole life be an act of worship. It is possible. When you eat, you can think, "I am feeding the Lord's temple." When you bathe, you can say, "I am washing the Lord's temple." When you sleep, you can think, "I am putting the Lord's temple to sleep." We can make our whole life like that: an offering. Offering away the fruits of our labor for the betterment of others keeps us easeful and peaceful, because we are not acting out of benefit for ourselves, but rather for the benefit of others. See your life as less of a journey towards a particular goal and see it as a dance. Be present. Everything is more perfect and whole than you know. Dance while the music is playing. Kiss life while you have lips to kiss. Play your part and do a good job. Anything weighing you down in this life is surely in your mind. Toss it overboard. You won't need any of it where we're going!

Om shanti shanti shanti

Acknowledgements

This book couldn't have been possible without the help of my sponsors and my being given permission to do anything and dream anything. Cal Clements and Jeremy Ayers are two men that truly helped me get to where I am today. To all of Athens's notable characters that helped me have the amazing story I've been so fortunate and lucky to have. To my father and mother, Ken Dean Ogletree and Kay Miller Turner, for their brilliant love that made me into the loving son I am today. To William Addison for his eternal guidance, love and friendship. I want to also acknowledge all the Yogis and Yoginis out there. Your work does not go unnoticed, nor is it in vain. To Victoria Butenko for educating me on how to go green for life! To Swami Satchidananda for his beauty that graced my life. To Ryokan, your life was poetry to my heart. To Hazrat Inayat Khan for initiating me into the temple of Sufism. To Hafiz for opening my heart so wide I fell into it laughing. To all the physicists that advance our species and expand our horizons. To Kofi Busia, Richard Freeman, Glen Black, and Rusty Wells for blessing me with their dedicated lives to Yoga. Special thanks to William Baxter for helping me finish the Yogi Residency and for being my first pre-order. To any and all spiritual aspirants on the path to samadhi, I bow to thee.

References

- *Green for Life*
- *Happy Yoga*
- *Healthy at 100*
- *Eat to Live*
- *Slaughter House*
- *Yoga Mala*
- The Yoga Sutras of Patañjali
- *The Art of Vinyasa*
- *A Brief History of Time*
- *Hyperspace*
- The yoga sutras
- *Peace is Every Step*
- *The Gift*
- *Dewdrops on a Lotus Leaf*
- *Beyond Words*
- *Roots of Yoga*
- yogajournal.com
- ashtangayoga.com
- 3ho.org
- merriam-webster.com
- ekhartyoga.com

Glossary

Asana – a posture adopted in performing hatha yoga

Ashram –a hermitage, monastic community, or other place of religious retreat

Ashtanga – a type of yoga based on eight principles and consisting of a series of poses executed in swift succession, combined with deep, controlled breathing

Asteya – non-stealing

Chakra – each of the centers of spiritual power in the human body, usually considered to be seven in number

Dandasana – staff pose

Dhyana – profound meditation that is the penultimate stage of yoga

Hari Om – Supreme Absolute Truth; "all that is"

Ishvara Pranidhana – surrendering to a higher source

Kaivalya Pada – liberation

Mantra – a word or sound repeated to aid concentration in meditation

Nadi Shodhana – Alternate Nostril Breathing

Niyamas – positive duties or observances; recommended activities and habits for healthy living, spiritual enlightenment and liberated state of existence

Om Shanti Shanti Shanti – peace

Pātañjalayogaśāstra – yoga attained by means of the eight auxiliaries

Prana – breath, considered as a life-giving force

Pratyahara – ingestion

Sadhana Pada – Yoga Sutras

Sadhana – daily spiritual practice

Sadhu – a holy man, sage, or ascetic

Samadhi – a state of intense concentration achieved through

meditation; final stage of yoga at which union with the divine is reached

Samadhi Pada – absorption

Samsara – the cycle of death and rebirth to which life in the material world is bound

Shamanism – a religion characterized by belief in an unseen world of gods, demons, and ancestral spirits responsive only to the shamans

Siddhi – complete understanding and enlightenment possessed by a siddha; a paranormal power possessed by a siddha

Surya Namaskara – Sun Salutations

Sutra – a rule or aphorism; scripture

Tapas – austerity; discipline

Vibhuti Pada – results

Vinyasa – movement between poses in yoga, typically accompanied by regulated breathing

Zen – a school of Buddhism emphasizing the value of meditation and intuition

One Last thing!

I'd like to thank everyone who has supported me by buying this book. If you feel inclined, please send me your thoughts, leave me your feedback, or write a review. Your support and your satisfaction with my work is deeply important to me.